Cancer Treatments

A complimentary approach

Roditch

Copyright

Contents

3

Introduction

Live your life in a health surplus to avoid most diseases and cure them.

This booklet is all about you. It gives you options that have helped many other people. The most important thing you can do when you have been diagnosed with cancer is to be in total control and know all your options before acting. After all your research, whatever you opt for—your oncologist, chemo, herbs, etc.—is of course your decision and your life. This booklet is all about you. It gives you options that have helped many other people. The most important thing you can do when you have been diagnosed with cancer is to be in total control and know all your options before acting. After all your research, whatever you opt for—your oncologist, chemo, herbs, etc.—is of course your decision and your life.

NOTE: When I say cure in this book, I mean that these treatments are known to either cure, slow down, reduce, and/or complement more conventional treatments of cancer.

It is a fact: there are cures for cancer that include natural medicines, pharmaceuticals, and a combination of both. Worldwide, many doctors are using holistic treatments to successfully cure cancer. Now there is a war going on between pharmaceutical companies and holistic doctors: over money and profits versus real, affordable cures. Most doctors only use radiation and chemotherapy supplied by Big Pharma. If you have been diagnosed with cancer, it is important to take a month and look at all your options. Do not rush or let an oncologist take over your health.

Among the things you can do, is go online and study what doctors and scientists are saying about cancer. Another is to find an oncologist who is happy to work with alternative therapies. This could be based on where you live, your bank balance, and whether you want to create your protocol or go to a clinic like the Hoxsey clinic in Mexico.

Luckily for you, there have been many scientific, research-based therapies developed over the last 20 years, that have been used by holistic doctors with real, verified success.

You have to choose between oncologists who sell expensive drugs and poisons and recommend eating pizza and ice cream, which is why you got cancer in the first place (doctors do not care about real health, i.e., organic food and herbs, etc.). or between a total healing program: spiritual, emotional, detox, raw organic foods, herbs, and supplements.

There may be times when your holistic doctor recommends chemotherapy in conjunction with holistic therapy; this is up to you. If you are full of fear, usually an oncologist will make that fear grow and kill you like an aboriginal pointing his bone. Don't ever listen to words that give you a sentence; there is always hope. Before you agree to "sign your health away" with an oncologist, ask to see their treatment records over the past 2 years. Total numbers of deaths, remissions, and cures If they won't show you, run.

Finally, the takeaway from all this is that modern science is finding new ways to cure cancer and can understand, using science, why certain protocols work, like Hoxsey and Gerson.

Free or inexpensive treatments

You should not worry too much about money if you want to treat your cancer naturally. Here is a list of things you can do that require you to have the willpower to change your life, your diet, and your belief system. Many of the things listed below are things you can do completely for free, like meditation, weight loss, exercise, and fasting, or things that require a change of diet, like eating organic food (or even growing your own) or juicing some of your vegetables, like carrots and beets. Eating more spices like ginger and turmeric Adding more herbs to your food, like garlic, basil, chili peppers, and lemongrass

Meditation

Meditation does not have to be an impossibility. There are a couple of easy ways to meditate and reduce mental activity and stress. One is mindfulness. Take your time, don't rush, enjoy the moment, and live in the moment, spending time with your kids, your parents, your wife, and in nature. Savor the taste of your food and the wind in your hair. The Dalai Lama said, "If you have a problem and it can be fixed, then fix it; if it cannot be fixed, worrying won't help." Another one is every time you catch your mind racing in fear, panic, evil thoughts, etc. STOP, breathe in slowly through your nose for 8 seconds, hold your breath for 8 seconds, and then, through a small hole in your lips, blow out slowly for 8 seconds, then hold for 4 seconds, and repeat 2 times as needed. When you hold your breath, it creates a relaxing state in your mind.

Food and Herbs

Apple Pectin: Absorbs toxins

Mushrooms

Mushrooms that grow on trees are very good for health and treat cancer, like cordyceps, shiitake, maitake, turkey tail, and Chaga. Hunt them down and include them in your diet. If you cannot find them to eat, they are available in supplement form.

Supplements

All these supplements are proven to help cure cancer.

Curcumin

Turmeric with a pinch of black pepper or Curcumin capsules which are much stronger.

Resveratrol

Grapes, dark chocolate, black raspberries, red wine, red grape juice, peanuts, pistachios, and peanut butter. Strawberries, blueberries, bilberries, cranberries, red currants, and mulberries.

Sulforaphane

Broccoli and broccoli sprouts, bok choy, and cabbage. Brussel sprouts. Kale and cabbage.

Green tea: Drink some every day.

Quercetin

Quercetin is a plant pigment (flavonoid). It is found in many plants and foods, such as red wine, onions, green tea, apples, berries, Ginkgo biloba, St. John's wort, American elder, and others. Buckwheat tea has a large amount of quercetin.

Vitamin C

Linus Pauling. Large intravenous doses of vitamin C for a month or more work. If you don't have access to injections straight away, build your vitamin C with vitamin C powder and vitamin C-rich fruits.

Boswellia

Indian Frankincense. good for brain tumors.

Artemisinin

Artemisia annua, sweet wormwood A Chinese herb that is also good for COVID-19

Lysine

Lysine is an amino acid, one of the building blocks of proteins. Lysine is classified as essential because the body can't make it. That means people must obtain it from their diets.

Found in raw pigs' pancreas. It is in protein-rich foods like meat, cheese, fish, eggs, and tofu. Yoghurt, Navy beans, salmon, chicken, tempeh, quinoa, soy milk, sardines, turkey, and lentils.

Manioc roots

Cassava root is particularly high in vitamin C, an important vitamin that acts as an antioxidant supports collagen production, and enhances immunity, among other benefits. Plus, it's rich in copper, a mineral necessary for neurotransmitter synthesis, energy production, iron metabolism, and more.

Soursop Leaves

Soursop and other plants have been shown to have promising compounds that could be used in the treatment of cancer. It is native to tropical and subtropical regions of the world, is extracted from the Annona muricata tree, and contains compounds that are particularly effective against cancer cells.

Salvestrol

Salvestrols are a type of phytochemical, a compound naturally found in plants that contribute to their color, taste, and smell. For instance, they give berries their red hue, veggies their bitter taste, and peppers their spicy taste. Salvestrols can be found in fruits and vegetables like Granny Smith apples, blueberries, strawberries, cranberries, avocados, broccoli,

Brussels sprouts, olives, cauliflower, cabbage, artichoke, basil, parsley, and rosemary.

Some of the common phytochemicals are:

Carotenoids in red, orange, yellow, and green plants may inhibit cancer growth and cardiovascular disease, and boost immunity.

Flavonoids in berries, apples, citrus, onions, soybeans, and coffee may fight inflammation and tumor growth.

Resveratrol in red wine, grapes, dark chocolate, and peanuts is associated with longevity in some animals.

Sleep

Sleep increases your body's ability to repair itself, reduces stress, and builds energy.

Skullcap

This medicinal plant references two herbs: American skullcap (Scutellaria lateriflora) and Chinese skullcap (Scutellaria baicalensis), with each being used to improve different conditions.

Research shows that Chinese skullcap extract is toxic to cancer cells, such as brain tumor cells, prostate cancer cells, and head and neck squamous cell carcinoma cell lines. Studies indicate that aqueous extracts suppressed the growth of lymphoma and myeloma cells.

Mistletoe

The liquid extract of the mistletoe plant has been used as an alternative method to treat cancer for close to a century. Mistletoe is one of the most widely researched naturopathic medicines prescribed for cancer patients in Europe. Numerous studies have shown mistletoe therapy may enhance cancer patient survival rates, improve quality of life, and reduce the side effects of chemotherapy and radiation.

Ginger

Some of the most studied actions of ginger are its analgesic and anti-inflammatory effects through the inhibition of NF-kB, COX-2, and 5-LOX (the major pathways and switches of inflammation mentioned previously). Ginger has also been shown to protect against cancer and to demonstrate a chemoprotective effect, meaning it protects the body from the side effects of chemotherapy.

Periwinkle flower (Catharanthus roseus)

A decades-long mystery centered on how the periwinkle transforms stemmadenine acetate into tabersonine and catharanthine, which ultimately couple to make the cancer-fighting compounds.

Vitamin B6

Epidemiologic and laboratory animal studies have suggested that the availability of vitamin B6 modulates cancer risk. How B6 mediates this effect is not known with any certainty, but it has been reported that high dietary vitamin B6 attenuates and low dietary vitamin B6 increases the risk of cancer.

Sources of Vitamin B6 are fish, beef liver and other organ meats, potatoes, and other starchy vegetables, fruit, and carrots.

Bone Broth

Bone broth builds a healthy immune system

Andrographis Paniculata

Andrographolide, a diterpenoid lactone isolated from the herbal plant Andrographis paniculata, is known to possess an anti-cancer effect. Andrographolide suppresses proliferation and triggers apoptosis in many types of cancer cells.

This is also approved for use in Thailand Hospitals for the treatment of covid-19 in the early stages. 180 MG a day for a week.

CBD Oil and leaves

CBD Oil or Blended Marijuana Leaves are a well-known cancer cure. The oil is a very convenient way to take it.

Eat the rainbow

Every day, eat the rainbow. All the different-colored vegetables and fruits will help you conquer cancer.

Microbiome

Probiotics and prebiotics—no antibiotics or GMO food Your immune system depends on a healthy gut. When you take a course of antibiotics, your microbiome is destroyed. You should think seriously before taking antibiotics. If you do need a course of antibiotics, you need to take probiotics for at least a month to overcome and fix the destruction. They come in pill form as well as in sour milk, sauerkraut, kimchee, and all fermented foods and drinks. When fighting cancer, you need an incredibly healthy microbiome, which means taking probiotics to the max every day.

Vitamin D - The sun

Vitamin D has become famous because it is a preventative against catching COVID-19. It boosts your immune system so much. Half an hour, naked in the midmorning sun, will give you a good dose.

Get in the sun, work, play, walk at the beach as often as you can.

Acupuncture

At specific locations on your skin, a professional uses tiny needles to provide acupuncture. According to studies, acupuncture may be useful in reducing chemotherapy-related nausea. In some cases, acupuncture can help cancer patients with their pain. If done by a trained professional using sterile needles, acupuncture is safe. Consult your healthcare provider for a list of reliable doctors. Consult your doctor before getting acupuncture if you're on blood thinners or have low blood counts. A similar method called acupressure involves applying light pressure to specific points, such as the wrist, to help with nausea relief.

Aromatherapy

Fragrant oils are used in aromatherapy to create a relaxing effect. When receiving a massage or taking a bath, you can apply oils to your skin that have been infused with aromas like lavender. To release their scents into the air, fragrant oils can also be heated. The benefits of aromatherapy may include pain, tension, and nausea relief. You can utilize aromatherapy on your own or have a professional execute it for you. Although oils applied to the skin can cause adverse responses, aromatherapy is safe. Avoid using a lot of lavender and tea tree oil on the skin if you have a malignancy that is estrogen sensitive, such as some breast cancers.

Cognitive behavioral therapy

A popular form of talk therapy is cognitive behavioral therapy (CBT). A mental health professional, such as a psychotherapist or therapist, works with you to view difficult events more clearly and react more effectively during a CBT session. CBT may be able to assist cancer patients with their sleep issues. You might get assistance from a CBT therapist or counselor in identifying and changing attitudes and behaviors that contribute to or exacerbate sleep issues with routines that encourage restful sleep. If you want to try CBT, ask your doctor for a recommendation to a specialist.

Exercise

Getting some exercise can help you control your symptoms both during and after cancer treatment. You may have less stress and exhaustion as a result of light exercise. Recent research suggests that an exercise regimen may lengthen cancer patients' lives and enhance their general quality of life. Before starting an exercise regimen, speak with your provider if you haven't been exercising frequently. Begin gradually and increase your exercise as you go. Work your way up to exercising for at least 30 minutes on most days of the week.

Hypnosis

A highly focused condition is hypnosis. A therapist may hypnotize you during a hypnotherapy session by speaking soothingly and assisting with relaxation. The therapist will then assist you in concentrating on objectives like managing your discomfort and lessening your tension. For those with cancer who are dealing with worry, discomfort, and anxiety, hypnosis may be beneficial. Additionally, if chemotherapy has previously made you feel ill, it may help minimize anticipatory nausea and vomiting that sometimes happen. Hypnosis is secure when carried out by a licensed therapist. But if you have a history of mental illness, let your therapist know.

Massage

Your massage therapist will knead your skin, muscles, and tendons while they work to calm you and ease any tension in your body. There are various massage techniques. Massage can be done lightly and gently or deeply and firmly. According to studies, massage therapy can be effective in reducing discomfort in cancer patients. Additionally, it might ease stress, weariness, and anxiety. If you work with a skilled massage therapist, massage can be safe. Many cancer treatment facilities have massage therapists on staff, or your doctor can recommend a massage therapist who frequently treats cancer patients. If you have extremely low blood counts, avoid getting a massage. Request that the massage therapist refrains from working on or near any tumors, radiation treatment sites, or surgical scars. Ask the massage therapist to use light pressure rather than deep massage if you have osteoporosis, cancer of the bones, or any other bone problems.

Meditation

When you concentrate your mind on a single image, sound, or idea, such as a positive thought, you are in a profound level of concentration. You might also practice deep breathing or relaxation techniques while meditating. Meditation may benefit cancer patients by reducing stress and anxiety and elevating mood. In general, meditation is secure. You can either do a class with an instructor or meditate on your own for a few minutes once or twice per day. Additionally, there are a ton of guided meditation applications and online courses accessible.

Music therapy

You might sing, play an instrument, or create lyrics while participating in music therapy sessions. You can take part in music therapy in a group setting or under the guidance of a qualified music therapist who will guide you through activities catered to your unique needs. In addition to reducing pain, worry, and tension, music therapy may also aid with nausea and vomiting management. Music talent is not necessary to participate in music therapy, which is safe. Certified music therapists work in a lot of hospitals.

Relaxation techniques

By using relaxation techniques, you can concentrate on lowering your stress levels and relaxing your body. Exercises in progressive muscle relaxation and visualization are two instances of relaxation methods. Relaxation practices might help to lessen anxiety and fatigue. Additionally, they might help cancer patients sleep better. Techniques for relaxation are secure. These exercises are typically guided by a therapist, but eventually, you may be able to perform them independently or with the aid of guided relaxation recordings.

Tai chi

Tai chi is a form of exercise that combines slow, deliberate breathing with soft motions. You can learn tai chi with a teacher, or you can do it alone by watching or reading books on the subject. Tai chi exercises could reduce stress. Tai chi is mostly risk-free. Since tai chi moves slowly, it doesn't demand a lot of physical strength, and the routines are simple to modify to your capabilities. However, consult your doctor before starting tai chi. Avoid any painful tai chi movements.

Yoga

Yoga mixes deep breathing with stretching exercises. You arrange your body in a variety of postures during a yoga session that calls for bending, twisting, and stretching. Yoga comes in a variety of forms, each with unique variants. People with cancer may find some respite from stress through yoga. Also proven to enhance sleep and lessen weariness is yoga. Before enrolling in a yoga class, ask your doctor for the name of a yoga instructor who has experience working with clients who have health issues, such as cancer. Avoid any painful yoga positions. An excellent instructor can provide safe alternatives for your positions.

Other relatively free things you can do

Coffee enemas

Coffee enemas are a good way to clean out your colon; this will detoxify your body. I am not sure how often you would need to do this. I have done it twice, and all sorts of chemicals came out looking like different colored powders and globs. I would try one coffee enema and see what comes out. After that, I prefer to wash my system out with water fasting or just eat a lot of juicy fruit for a day and drink loads of water, and it will eventually be released through my bowels in a whoosh. Cleaning them out from the stomach to the butt

Detox Fasting

Studies have shown that water fasting could have health benefits. For example, it may lower the risk of some chronic diseases and stimulate autophagy, a process that helps your body break down and recycle old parts of your cells.

Detox with Moringa and Cilantro

Cilantro is easy to buy. Moringa is an Asian tree. You can eat or juice the leaves. It is a very powerful plant.

Rebound on a small trampoline

When you jump you activate your lymph system. Your lymph system helps clean your body. It is important to do at least 30 minutes a day on a small trampoline to get your lymph system flowing.

Trypsin and chymotrypsin dissolve protein coating on cancer cells

Protein-dissolving enzymes (trypsin and chymotrypsin) - are derived from a pig pancreas because it is very similar to that of the human pancreas, thus making it much more capable of dissolving the fibrin coating that surrounds tumors than vegetable-derived enzymes. Using systemic enzymes as part of an overall cancer healing program

Clean Water

Clean water, PH neutral, is essential for curing cancer.

Organic Raw Foods

Most non-organic foods are sprayed with Roundup. Roundup has glyphosate in it. A lot of foods are now GMO, which also have a lot of glyphosates in it. This is a well-known cancer-causing substance. Also, when you cook your food, you lose vitamins, enzymes, and other nutrients. When you have cancer, you need to get the maximum benefit out of your food that you can. There are many vegetables, and of course, fruit, that you can eat raw. And organic food will heal your body.

Some Herbs - Do your research for more

Turmeric - Curcumin Dr Thomas Iodi.

Wormwood, Ginger, Cilantro, Moringa Leaves, Soursop Leaves, Cayenne Pepper, Marijuana Leaves, Boswellia, Andrographis.

Bitter herbs include ginger, turmeric, milk thistle, cilantro, dandelion greens

Iodine

Cancer starts with iodine deficiencies just as it does with low oxygenation of tissues, with no one looking into the fact that low iodine and low oxygenation of tissues are directly related. Doctors are still scratching their heads, wondering why cancer rates have been exploding, but do not pay attention to doctors who have seen over 90 percent deficiency rates among their patients and reports of other doctors seeing the same.

Activated charcoal

Taking one activated charcoal tablet with a few glasses of water helps detox your body. There are mixed views about the value of using this product.

Lose Weight

Being overweight is normally not healthy and increases your risk of cancer. If you lose weight

Using the keto diet, you will also benefit from reducing your blood sugar levels; remember, cancer loves sugar.

Universal God

I believe in a universal God. This helps me feel connected to other people, animals, nature, the earth, and the universe. It is important to feel that you are not alone when you have cancer.

Praying, meditating, and talking to the universal God usually bring many benefits. The Universal God is represented in all religions and spiritual beliefs, whether religious or not. If you wish to make contact, it is up to you if you want to go within to find your Universal God or without, to experience the fellowship of religions like Hinduism, Christianity, Islam, and Buddhism. I think if you are living in countries like America, Australia, and England and you are not a Christian, it is important to understand that God is not a religion. God is the universal energy that permeates everything, including humans, with whom we need to communicate daily.

Brassica and Cruciferous Vegetables

Cruciferous vegetables: broccoli, cabbage, kale, radish, chard, cauliflower, bok choy, kohlrabi, Brussels sprouts, watercress, collards, mustard greens, turnips, pepper, daikon root, and arugula.

Sprouts

Sprouted seeds are full of cancer-fighting nutrients like sulforaphane in Broccoli seeds and watercress seeds.

Fruit and Vegetable Juicing

Wheatgrass, beetroot, celery, carrot, pineapple, and more

Essential Oils

Frankincense oil is particularly good for brain tumors.

Other essential oils will help you too. Turmeric, Clary sage, citrus, orange, mandarin, and carrot

Cheap Protocols

Budwig Diet

Flaxseed oil and cottage cheese.

People on the diet eat a mixture of flaxseed oil, cottage cheese, and honey multiple times per day. Typically, this "Budwig mixture" is made by combining cottage cheese and flaxseed oil in a 2:1 ratio, alongside a small amount of honey.

You're encouraged to eat at least 2 ounces (60 mL) of flaxseed oil and 4 ounces (113 grams) of cottage cheese per day. This concoction should be prepared fresh at each meal and eaten within 20 minutes. High-fiber foods are also recommended, including fruits and vegetables. Conversely, you should avoid sugar, refined grains, processed meat, and other processed foods.

Lysine diet

Raw pancreas pig, raw cow liver, 8 raw eggs a day with chili. This is from Dr. William Donald Kelley.

B17

Apple and apricot kernel seeds,

Laetrile. Apple and Apricot seeds, 20mg of Vitamin B17, 5 kernels 10 times a day for a week then 10 a day. Also in berries, grains beans, and leafy green vegetables.

Homeopathic - what have you got to lose?

Homeopathic medicine has been around for a long time. It is well known the royal family in England use them.

714X

Developed by the researcher and biologist Gaston Naessens in the 1970s, 714X is categorized as an immuno-modulator health product aiming to either support a weak immune system or slow down an overactive one. It intends to restore the body's immune defenses without causing side effects.

Angustura Vera and other homeopathic cures for cancer

Ketogenic diet

The ketogenic diet is a very low-carb, high-fat diet that shares many similarities with the Atkins and low-carb diets.

It involves drastically reducing carbohydrate intake and replacing it with fat. This reduction in carbs puts your body into a metabolic state called ketosis.

When this happens, your body becomes incredibly efficient at burning fat for energy. It also turns fat into ketones in the liver, which can supply energy to the brain.

Ketogenic diets can cause significant reductions in blood sugar and insulin levels. This, along with the increased ketones, has some health benefits. This reduction in sugar helps fight cancer because cancer loves sugar. Also, weight loss improves your health dramatically.

Free protocols - Things to stop and let go

All sugar - try stevia

Stress - Relax and meditate. Make your mind peaceful

Junk Food - None,

Chemo - unless with holistic doctor

Non-GMO food - Eat only organic

Food grown in bio sludge - eat organic

Stop cooking all your food eat some raw - salads, sprouts, juices, smoothies etc.

Don't use 5g networks on your phone. Use qi technology to protect you.

More expensive protocols

Dr. Burzynski

https://www.burzynskiclinic.com/

Innovative and cutting-edge Precision Personalized Cancer Therapy

Medical expertise based on over 40 years of clinical experience and research

Our goal is to provide sophisticated cancer care utilizing a personalized and precision-targeted immunotherapy approach.

Our personalized cancer therapy utilizes an understanding of each patient's cancer genetic and immunotherapy makeup to unravel the biology of their cancer and to identify effective treatment strategies using targeted therapies and immunotherapies that are aimed at specific genes or proteins that are found only in cancer cells or their environment.

TREATING CANCER SINCE 1977

Established in 1977, the Burzynski Clinic has grown to be a nationally and internationally recognized cancer center that provides cutting-edge cancer treatments.

For over 40 years, Dr. Burtynsky's cancer research and patient care have been inspired by the philosophy of the physician Hippocrates: "First, not harm." Therefore, our approach to treatment is "personalized" to maximize effectiveness and minimize side effects for each cancer patient.

Dr Rath - Books

https://www.drrathresearch.org/

Dr Rath's discoveries and our research set up new therapeutic directions and present a real chance to control cancer, all of which had not been possible with conventional medical approaches. We have demonstrated that a specific combination of natural substances (vitamins, amino acids, polyphenols, and other micronutrients) working in biological synergy can successfully control critical aspects of malignancy in our body, such as:

Curtail metastasis (the spread of cancer to other organs)

Inhibit tumor growth

Decrease tumor angiogenesis (formation of new blood vessels feeding tumors)

Trigger natural death of cancer cells through apoptosis.

Gerson Therapy

https://gerson.org/gerpress/the-gerson-therapy/

The Gerson TherapyTM is a natural treatment that activates the body's extraordinary ability to heal itself through an organic, plant-based diet, raw juices, coffee enemas, and natural supplements.

The Gerson TherapyTM, with its whole-body approach to healing, naturally reactivates your body's magnificent ability to heal itself - with no harmful side effects. This powerful, natural treatment boosts the body's immune system to heal cancer, arthritis, heart disease, allergies, and many other degenerative diseases. Dr. Max Gerson developed the Gerson TherapyTM in the 1930s, initially as a treatment for his debilitating migraines and eventually as a treatment for degenerative diseases such as skin tuberculosis, diabetes, and, most famously, cancer.

The Hoxsey Therapy

https://www.hoxseybiomedical.com/

Biomedical Centre Mexico Tijuana - Liz Jones

If you have cancer or know someone who does, you already understand the physical and psychological toll that it takes on a person. The symptoms of the disease are both painful and distressing. Conventional treatments do not always work and often cause serious side effects.

Modern medicine has made incredible progress in improving human health. However, conventional cancer treatment is often very painful to the patient and is not always effective. Fortunately, there are now alternative therapies that can offer great results without the problems that are associated with mainstream therapies.

Bio-Medical Center specializes in alternative therapies for cancer and a wide variety of illnesses and conditions. Patients with multiple sclerosis, emphysema, and other problems have all benefited from these remedies. Regardless of the illness being treated, the doctors here believe that helping the patient maintain a high quality of life is an essential part of any cure.

Intravenous Vitamin C

Discovered by Dr. Linus Pauling.

With Intravenous vitamin C, you must make your mind up like all the others. It should help a lot. But not your sole attack.

Essiac Tea

This is a popular treatment. It is an American Indian recipe that is made up of burdock root, sheep sorrel, slippery elm, and Indian rhubarb root.

Hyperbaric Chamber

Pump your cells full of cancer-killing oxygen

Hyperbaric chamber therapy, otherwise known as hyperbaric oxygen therapy (HBOT), is a medical treatment used to help boost the body's natural healing processes.

Historically, hyperbaric oxygen therapy was first used in the U.S. in the early 1900s. Later, it was used to treat decompression sickness, a hazard of scuba diving. Today, HBOT is prescribed and supervised medically by institutions such as Mayo Clinic, and it may even be covered by insurance (depending on the condition it's used to treat).

Hydrotherapy

Hydrotherapy uses water and temperature such as hot/cold baths, saunas, whirlpools, wraps, colonics, enemas, etc., as a method to promote healing. Various forms of water therapy have been used for centuries in the treatment of disease and injury by many cultures including those of ancient Rome, China, and Japan.

BCE5 - Curaderm for Skin Cancer

This was discovered in Australia by Dr. Bill Cham when animals with eye cancer rubbed themselves up against a Devil's Apple Tree.

From a scientific perspective, Professor Dr. Bill Cham has achieved a scientist's dream. From laboratory experiments, he has discovered and identified substances in plant material that showed anticancer properties when investigated in test tubes. He then proceeded to show that these substances, now known as BEC, were killing cancer cells and, most importantly, why BEC was not killing normal cells. Finally, he critically evaluated the results of his experiments and applied them to the treatment of human skin cancer. The outcome is now history, and treatment for non-melanoma skin cancer is available to the public.

These events were not fortuitous; they were achieved by tenacious, accurate, and responsible work in which lateral thinking was essential. His lateral thinking was fed by his background training at highly regarded universities worldwide. He has a degree in chemistry, a degree in biochemistry, and holds a doctorate in the school of medicine, which is exactly the recipe for mastering drug development and taking it to clinical application. His achievements in the scientific field are evidenced by the recognition of his work worldwide and the fact that, currently, many scientists are applying and extending his observations in the search for a treatment for terminal internal cancers.

http://www.curadermbec5.com/

Removing Amalgam fillings that have mercury.

Mercury, as we all know, is a highly toxic heavy metal, as mentioned in this post on the leaky gut syndrome. Even low levels of exposure can lead to a variety of adverse health conditions. Still, it continues to be used as a major component in silver amalgam fillings. While you may think your fillings are stable and solid and are not leaching into your system, any amount of friction can cause the fillings to release small amounts of Mercury gas. This gas may subsequently be absorbed into the body, resulting in mercury toxicity. The connection between "silver amalgam" fillings and cancer was first discovered in Europe, and many countries within the European Union have since banned or greatly restricted their use. Unfortunately, the United States has yet to follow suit, and mercury-contaminated "silver amalgam" fillings are still the most common type of filling used by dentists in the US.

Acupuncture

Acupuncture has proven effective in treating and supporting different facets of cancer and cancer treatments.

Infrared Sauna

Sauna is not a recent invention of mankind. The cradle of the sauna is far from the luxurious spas of today. Ancient civilizations from all parts of the world once made use of rudimentary facilities to raise body temperature (hyperthermia) to promote profuse sweating, aware that this powerful mechanism could activate healing processes in the body.

The healing effects of a sauna are mainly derived from the activation of the parasympathetic system.

Science has further proven several benefits of the regular use of saunas and in particular the use of the infrared sauna, which uses infrared radiation (or light) to increase temperature. It also has more therapeutic effects when compared to steam.

Deep detoxification

An integrative approach to treating cancer will never be complete without a detoxification program. Among the different ways to eliminate waste from our bodies, sweat plays a key role.

It has been said that the skin is the main detoxification organ in our body. Heavy metals, phenols, phthalates, medications of chronic use, and many other cancer-causing chemicals are expelled through our pores when we sweat.

Pulsed Electromagnetic Field Therapy (PEMF or PEMT

Pulsed electromagnetic field therapy is a non-invasive, painless treatment that works by emitting a pulsating, varying intensity, and frequency electromagnetic field from a solenoid placed around the patient. Pulsed electromagnetic field therapy was approved by the FDA in 1979 for the treatment of non-union fractures, following a Columbia University study supported by NASA, and has recently gained popularity in the United States (even appearing as a segment on the Dr. Oz Show). The value of pulsed electromagnetic field therapy has been shown to cover a wide range of conditions, with well-documented trials carried out by hospitals, rheumatologists, physiotherapists, and neurologists. PEMF was widely used and had great success in the 19th and early 20th centuries. These primitive electromagnetic therapeutic devices were used by both medical doctors and non-allopathic health practitioners.

PEMF therapies may be one approach to enhancing the value of existing treatments for cancer. There may be benefits related to improving healthy oxygen circulation, promoting the growth of healthy cells, and improving the quality of breathing, which are of particular benefit to individuals with lung cancer. PEMF therapy may also help with the pain. Cancer often brings with it one or more of four different types of pain.

Wellbeing

Spiritual and emotional

Always stay positive. Clear your mind of negative thoughts about cancer, especially any from your oncologist.

God is a universal term for spiritual energy, Universal laws, mathematical structures, entwining the universe, and all life. Get involved and get connected with the FORCE.

Meditation, swimming, yoga, prayer, mindfulness, faith, trust, sleep and walking in the forest. There are many ways to calm your mind and relax. You need to reduce your stress, and your mental chatter and be positive about your treatments, which may include old conventional, new conventional, and natural treatments and solutions

Evox Therapy

Releasing negative emotions using Evox therapy

Recall Healing

https://www.recallhealing.com/

Hawaiian way of forgiving yourself. Please forgive me, I love you, and thank you.

A list of Doctors and Healers

All these doctors and health practitioners have something special to say and offer. Dr. Brownstein, the Health Ranger (Mike Adams), and Dr. Sircus, Dr. Axe I know well and respect them a lot.

When you have been diagnosed with cancer you need to stop as much as you can, take a deep breath, make a lot of notes, and make a plan that feels good. You will have to pick your way through this mini-book and especially the doctors over a quiet, peaceful week. This is the secret to health. Don't let your monkey mind distract you from saving your life or the life of a loved

Dr. Sircus

www.drsircus.com

Dr. Martin Goldstein

https://drmarty.com/

Dr. Thomas Seyfried

https://tomseyfried.com/

Dr. Yanigasawa

https://riordanclinic.org/speaker-archive/atsuo-yanagisawa-md-phd/

Dr. Homer Lim

https://cancerhealerph.com/homerlim/

Dr. Rengasamy

http://www.sahamm.org/the-scary-big-c-cancer/

Dr. Gaston Cornu-Labat

https://www.healthgrades.com/physician/dr-gaston-cornu-labat-yhs4r

Dr. Max Gerson

https://gerson.org/gerpress/dr-max-gerson/

Dr. Brownstein

www.drbrownstein.com

The Health Ranger

www.naturalnews.com

Dr. Keith Scott Mumby

https://alternative-doctor.com/

Dr. Axe

www.draxe.com

Burzynski Clinic

https://www.burzynskiclinic.com/

Dr. Rath

https://www.drrathresearch.org/

https://www.drrathresearch.org/research/projects/cancer

https://www.dr-rath-foundation.org/cellular-medicine/

Hoxsey Therapy

https://www.hoxseybiomedical.com/

Dr. Cham

http://www.curadermbec5.com/

Dr. Joseph Mercola

https://www.mercola.com/

Dr. Jonathon Wright

https://tahomaclinic.com/

Dr. Patrick Quillin

https://patrickquillin.com/

Dr. John Beard

https://www.cancerfightingstrategies.com/enzymes-for-cancer.html

https://www.healingcancernaturally.com/trophoblastic-theory-of-cancer.html

https://alternative-doctor.com/dr-john-beard/

Bob Wright

https://www.cancertutor.com/bob_wright/

Dr. Buttar

https://www.drbuttar.com/nine-cancer-cures-that-the-medical-mafia-doesnt-want-you-to-know-about/

Dr. Lewis Thomas

https://www.nytimes.com/1993/12/04/obituaries/lewis-thomas-whose-essays-clarified-the-mysteries-of-biology-is-dead-at-80.html

Shu Funase

https://jackiebye.com/family/celebrating-our-freedoms-what-about-medical-freedom-with-treating-cancer/

Dr. Tony Jimenez

https://hope4cancer.com/about-us/our-doctors/dr-tony-jimenez-m-d/

Bob Wright

https://www.cancertutor.com/bob_wright/

Sayer Ji

https://www.greenmedinfo.com/

Joel Salatin

http://www.polyfacefarms.com/joels-bio/

Dr. Yu cheng kuo

http://innovationinfo.org/index.php/journal/editorial_board_member/Dr-Yu-Cheng-Kuo

Dr. Baylock

https://www.blaylockreport.com/

Dr. Sunil Pai

https://sanjevani.net/our-center/sunil-pai-md/

Dr. Suzanne Humphries

https://medium.com/@visualvaccines/why-dr-suzanne-humphries-an-anti-vaccine-activist-is-lying-to-you-about-measles-ce446d0a7e0f

https://www.facebook.com/drsuzanne

Dr. Rigvr

https://www.dr-adem.com/rigvir/

Dr. Hassami

https://www.bumrungrad.com/en/centers/horizon-cancer-treatment-center-bangkok-thailand

Dr. Palevsky

https://www.northportwellnesscenter.com/practitioner/lawrence-palevsky/about

Del Bigtree

https://www.bitchute.com/channel/okiFK5CwQrZS/

Dr. Chris Motley

https://www.doctormotley.com/

Dr. Billy Demoss

https://demosschiropractic.com/

Dr. Tenpenny

https://www.drtenpenny.com/

Dr. Badakashan

https://www.cancercenterforhealing.com/bita-badakhshan-md/

Dr. Thomas Lodi

https://drthomaslodi.com/

Dr. Chilkov

https://www.integrativecanceranswers.com/dr-nalini-chilkov/

Dr. Simoncini

https://www.cancertutor.com/simoncini/

Dr. Scott Bell

http://www.robertscottbell.com/

Dr. Billy Demoss

https://demosschiropractic.com/

Cilla Whatcott

https://www.gofundme.com/f/cilla039s-alternative-cancer-treatment

Dr. Farley

https://drjamesfarley.com/articles/proper-immune-function-covid-19/

Dr. Ben Johnson

https://drbennaturals.com/who-is-dr-ben-johnson/

Dr. Homer Lim

https://cancerhealerph.com/homerlim/

9 Cancer Cures You Might Want to Know!

Cures mean partial or total solutions

Turmeric

Most turmeric sold in America suffers from the high lead content and a high count of microbes. By purchasing cheap turmeric, you could be increasing the heavy metal toxins and bacteria that you consume, driving cancer cells. Do the exact opposite! Find an organic turmeric tincture that contains the phytonutrient curcumin, and you can build natural immunity.

Hemp seed oil

An essential oil is created by cold-pressing the seeds of the Cannabis sativa (hemp) plant, and it is legal to buy it in health food stores across the country in the US! It has a very high concentration of necessary fatty acids but is devoid of the hallucinogenic THC element found in marijuana. It is considered a "superfood" because of its special ratio of omega-3 to omega-6 essential fatty acids and because it contains up to 5% pure GLA, which is higher than in spirulina. It is a member of the achene family of fruits. Hemp seed oil has been used for thousands of years in elixirs and medicinal teas to give an anti-mutagenic effect that guards against genetic damage caused by free radicals and/or radiation.

Reishi mushrooms

Reishi doesn't appear in packages or on salads at your neighborhood regular grocery store. Check out the supplements and dried powders, which are typically marketed as capsules, in health food stores. For more than 2,000 years,

Reishi has been utilized in the Far East to treat a wide range of illnesses. They are referred to as "mushrooms of immortality" in China. Reishi is supposed to be consumed over an extended period and has been connected to enhanced nerve health and blood pressure reduction! Reishi mushrooms may be used to treat diabetes and cancer, but don't tell the hospital administrators or the local newspaper because they may have to report you to the Medical Mafia. The oncologists' cash registers stop ringing, and they send you home to live when you start talking about significant polysaccharides and saponins that reduce cell multiplication in malignant lungs.

Melatonin

Hello, free-radical scavengers! Did you know that as you sleep, you can protect yourself from free-radical damage? It is real. Melatonin is a versatile, antioxidant-rich chemical ever since it was discovered more than 50 years ago. Because it has 200 percent higher antioxidant potential than vitamin E, an extensive experimental study has proven its crucial function in the body's defense against multiple cell-damaging free radicals. Melatonin is superior to glutathione and vitamins C and E in reducing oxidative damage. It combats conditions like cancer and cardiovascular disease that are linked to free radicals. Although the brain naturally creates melatonin, it's typical to need supplements if you have diabetes, is at risk for developing it, or are over 55. Consult a naturopath!

Real spring water

Without additional fluoride (with an average pH level of 8.8), if you're battling cancer, you're probably desperate to change the pH of your body. Almost every dietitian on the planet will advise you to eat a lot of unprocessed, organic fruits and vegetables as well as to drink a lot of water, preferably pure spring water, to help the body become more alkaline.

Baking soda

Yes, the affordable variety that is available at most stores. Simply mix a teaspoon with a glass of water each day to help alkalize your body, which will prevent cancer from ever trying to live. When your body is not acidic and your cells have enough oxygen, cancer cannot survive. Because the use of baking soda is so straightforward, you'll never hear a doctor or oncologist recommend it because the AMA, FDA, and FTC will shut them down. Selling baking soda and the cancer cure will not bring in any money for the mafia-style medical industry.

Organic garlic cloves

More than 200 biologically active components fight off infections! Ornithine decarboxylase is a specific enzyme that the "bad guys" (mutated cells) employ to reproduce. By inhibiting this enzyme, you can cut off the adversary's "supply lines." If cancer cells lacked a source of energy, how much simpler would it be to treat them?

Apricot seed kernels

Efficient alternative cancer treatment is carelessly hidden by the apricot seed "cyanide" debate. Numerous studies show that apricot seeds can effectively treat cancer without causing any side effects. What if the "cyanide" that terrifies you is actually the type that KILLS CANCER and NOT YOU? Let the medical mafia not deter you from a long life!

Cannabis sativa

In 2700 BC, the "Father of Chinese Medicine" identified marijuana's therapeutic benefits. Ancient civilizations, including the Egyptians, Persians, and even Greeks, used medical marijuana throughout history. Because the DEA categorizes it unreasonably as a Schedule I narcotic and thus deters potential patients and physicians, mainstream medicine in the USA is particularly reluctant to realize this.

Some Science

47

Cells have a protein coating

Cancer cells are coated with protein, which makes it hard for the immune system to kill them. Trypsin and chymotrypsin can dissolve the protein. It is available from raw pig pancreas and other sources.

And another way Over 100 years ago, Dr. John Beard at the University of Edinburgh discovered that the body's primary mechanism for destroying cancer is contained in pancreatin, a secretion from the pancreas that includes enzymes for digesting protein. among other things. Dr. Beard presented papers to show recoveries using pancreatin to attack the malignancy without the toxic side effects on other functions of the body.

(https://attackingcancer.org/enzyme-therapy-the-century-old-cancer-treatment/)

Hypoxia-inducible factors, or HIFs

Cancer cells in a growing tumor can adapt to oxygen deprivation by hijacking these HIFs

For example, HIF turns on a protein called VEGF to induce new blood vessels, and multiple VEGF inhibitory drugs are now used to fight cancer. (https://blog.dana-farber.org/insight/2019/11/cancer-and-oxygen-whats-the-connection/)

Sugar

Cancer likes sugar. It is good to avoid all sugar. Losing weight helps fight cancer. The Ketogenic diet helps lose weight AND reduce blood sugar levels.

You might have heard that sugar causes cancer or makes it grow faster. In some ways, this makes sense. Every cell in your body uses blood sugar (glucose) for energy. But cancer cells use about 200 times more energy than normal cells. Tumors that start in the thin, flat (squamous) cells in your lungs gobble up even more glucose. They need huge amounts of sugar to fuel their growth.

The idea that cancer cells thrive on sugar has been around at least since the 1924 publication of Dr. Otto Warburg's paper, On the Metabolism of Tumors. Warburg was a Nobel Prize-winning cell biologist who hypothesized that cancer growth was caused when cancer cells converted glucose into energy through glycolysis in the presence of oxygen. The Warburg Effect, present in the majority of cancers, is another name for aerobic glycolysis. 1 This was an interesting assertion, in part because we know that healthy cells make energy by converting pyruvate into oxygen. The pyruvate is oxidized within a healthy cell's mitochondria. Since cancer cells don't oxidize pyruvate, Warburg thought cancer must be considered a mitochondrial dysfunction.

Oxygen

Cancer thrives in a low-oxygen environment. Lots of oxygen can help fight cancer. Time in a Hyperbaric chamber can do this.

Mitochondria

Mitochondria are membrane-bound cell organelles (mitochondrion, singular) that generate most of the chemical energy needed to power the cell's biochemical reactions. Chemical energy produced by the mitochondria is stored in a small molecule called adenosine triphosphate (ATP). Mitochondria contain their small chromosomes. Juicing fruit and vegetables is one way to increase the energy of the Mitochondria and kill cancer.

Inflammation encourages cancer to grow

Ginger and Turmeric are good for reducing inflammation.

B17

How Does B17 Kill Cancer Cells?

Firstly, be aware that vitamin B17 is made up of two molecules of glucose (a sugar), one molecule of hydrocyanic acid (hydrogen cyanide), and one molecule of benzaldehyde (an analgesic/painkiller). This is a simple description of how B17 kills cancer. Enzymes are used by our bodies for a variety of processes. Rhodanese is the name of one of these enzymes. Except for the areas of our body where cancer cells are located, it is present in large amounts everywhere else. A novel enzyme manifests itself at the cancer site when cancer is present. The name of it is beta-glucosidase. Beta-glucosidase, which is not present elsewhere in our bodies besides where cancer cells are, and rhodanese are both present everywhere in our bodies but not where cancer cells are.

When vitamin B17 enters the body, the enzyme rhodanese immediately breaks it down. It transforms it into thiocyanate and benzoic acid, two by-products. The nourishment of healthy cells can benefit from both byproducts. In excess, these byproducts are removed through urination. The rhodanese starts converting B17 the moment it enters your body. In the body, the B17 lasts for about 80 minutes. The body excretes more than 80% of the vitamin in question in just 4 hours. Providing the patient with proper nutritional support, doses of vitamins and minerals, and other potent natural substances is the typical metabolic approach to vitamin B17 therapy.

There is no rhodanese to break down vitamin B17 when it interacts with a cancer cell that is destroying tissue. There is only beta-glucosidase left in the body right now. One molecule of benzaldehyde and one molecule of hydrogen cyanide are synergistically combined when B17 and beta-glucosidase come into contact. As a result, a toxin is produced that kills the cancer cell. When beta-glucosidase is present, vitamin B17 selectively targets and kills cancer cells.

Cyanide-not as scary as you think

The word "cyanide" can now be a little frightening. You've probably read, as have I, that "cyanide" is bad. Not all cyanide compounds, though, are poisonous. Humans are constantly exposed to cyanide because it is found in more than 1,200 different types of food, is released into the air when materials like plastic and cigarette smoke are burned, is present in the chemical used to develop photographs, and is also present in the air we breathe. It is also used to make textiles, plastic, and paper in addition to being present in cyanide. In other words, everyday activities including breathing air, touching the earth, drinking water, and eating food expose you to cyanide.

B17 contains no "free hydrogen cyanide" either. Hydrochlorine must be created. Do you recall when we talked about the enzyme beta-glucosidase? This enzyme is the only one that can convert vitamin B17 into hydrogen cyanide. There won't be any beta-glucosidase if there are no cancer cells present.

Without beta-glucosidase, hydrogen cyanide generated from vitamin B17 cannot be produced. Is there a different way to produce hydrogen cyanide? I don't think so, but even if there were, the production would be so minuscule that any hazardous effects would be minimal at best. The drugs used in chemotherapy are thousands of times more poisonous than B17.

However, vitamin B17 contains the cyanide radical (CN). I'd like to ask you this. Are you a fan of strawberries? Did you ever consume them? Well, if you consumed them, you did consume that cyanide radical. Strawberries and vitamin B12 both contain it. Have you ever heard of someone consuming cyanide after consuming vitamin B12 or strawberries? I didn't.

RIGVR

What are the side effects of Rigvir®? Other than fatigue and sleepiness, some patients feel a little feverish (up to 99.5 °F). This is a good thing because it means their immune system is up and running.

What types of tumors does Rigvir® treat? Rigvir® can be used to fight solid tumors only. This means it cannot help fight such malignancies as leukemia, myeloma, and lymphomas. You will find the complete list of Rigvir®-sensitive tumors later in the article.

Can Rigvir® be combined with other treatments? Yes, Rigvir® can be combined with chemotherapy and radiotherapy as well as used as a monotherapy. Please note, however, that Rigvir® cannot be recommended as a preventive measure or in non-cancer cases.

Chemotherapy

Chemotherapy medications disturb cells to work. Varied medications have different impacts on specific malignancies and target various growth phases. Drugs used in chemotherapy are unable to distinguish between diseased and healthy cells, which can have negative effects on the patient. Cancer cells normally do not recover from the effects of chemotherapy, although healthy cells frequently do.

Here is a list of some of the most common chemotherapy medications for use during cancer treatment.

Alkylating agents

These were among the first cancer therapies, and they are being utilized often today. They function by causing damage to the DNA within cells, which stops the cells from dividing. Although they are useful against many different types of cancer, they are most potent against slow-growing tumors.

Antimetabolites

These medications function by making cells appear to require growth. After devouring them, the cell gradually starves to death. These drugs only function during phases of a cell's development cycle.

Plant alkaloids

Plant alkaloids are organic compounds that stop malignant cells from reproducing and proliferating. They can function at any time during a cell's growth cycle, but stages are when they perform best.

Anti-tumor antibiotics

These medications treat infections differently than antibiotics. They function by breaking off DNA strands, which stops the cell from dividing.

Some Chemotherapies from nature

Taxol

Taxol originally came from the Pacific yew tree (Taxus brevifolia). Now, doctors use synthetic versions. What is Taxol?

Taxol is an anti-cancer ("antineoplastic" or "cytotoxic") chemotherapy drug. Taxol is classified as a "plant alkaloid," a "taxane" and an "antimicrotubule agent."

Taxol is used for the treatment of breast, ovarian, lung, bladder, prostate, melanoma, esophageal, as well as other types of solid tumor cancers. It has also been used in Kaposi's sarcoma.

Epirubicin - a drug from the soil

Epirubicin, a compound that was isolated from a soil bacterium called Streptomyces, is one of those little elements of the natural world we often ignore. Epirubicin is used in combination with other medications to treat breast cancer in patients who have had surgery to remove the tumor. Epirubicin is in a class

of medications called anthracyclines. It works by slowing or
stopping the growth of cancer cells in your body

Alternatives to Chemotherapy

Chemotherapy is an effective and widely used cancer treatment that kills rapidly dividing cells, including healthy tissue. Because of this, chemotherapy can cause serious side effects. There is a slowly growing range of alternative treatments that may have fewer risks, but they also come with several limitations.

Alternative therapies to chemotherapy include photodynamic therapy, laser therapy, immunotherapy, targeted therapy, and hormone therapy. Individuals should discuss possible treatments with medical professionals to establish which treatment may be most beneficial for them.

Photodynamic Therapy

In photodynamic therapy (PDT), medications that kill cancer cells are activated by light from a laser or other light source. PDT is frequently used by medical professionals as a local therapy to treat a particular body part. PDT has been authorized by the Food and Drug Administration (FDA) to treat a variety of malignancies and precancers, including:

actinic keratosis advanced cutaneous T-cell lymphoma

Barrett's esophagus

basal cell skin cancer

non-small cell lung cancer

stage 0 squamous cell skin cancer

If certain malignancies start to obstruct the throat or airways, doctors may also employ PDT to treat their symptoms. PDT can only be used to treat cancers that are in the lining of organs and cavities, immediately under the skin, or on the skin itself. PDT entails the individual taking a photosensitizer medication, either orally, topically on the skin, or straight into a vein. Cancer cells absorb the medication in 24-72 hours, after which time doctors expose them to light. Light and the medication combine to produce oxygen, which kills cancer cells.

Laser therapy

In laser therapy, a physician uses a concentrated light beam to heat and remove precancerous growths and tiny tumors. They can also use it to address symptoms like bleeding and to reduce tumors that block parts of the digestive tract. After surgery, surgeons may use a laser to shut nerve endings or lymphatic veins, which lessens pain and swelling and prevents the spread of tumor cells. In PDT, the photosensitizing agent may also be activated by lasers.

Immunotherapy

A biological therapy called immunotherapy aids in boosting a person's natural defenses to manage and defeat cancer. Immunotherapy comes in several different ways. It functions by enhancing the immunological response, boosting immune cells, and instructing the immune system to identify and target cancer cells.

Targeted Therapy

With targeted therapy, medical professionals treat each patient specifically rather than applying a blanket strategy. These treatments either consist of monoclonal antibodies that attach to targets on cancer cells or tiny molecule medicines that can quickly enter cells.

Hormone Therapy

Certain cancers rely on hormones to grow, thus treating them to block or alter these hormones may prevent cancer from spreading. Some breast, endometrial, and prostate cancers that depend on sex hormones to proliferate are generally treated with hormone therapy.

Some more ideas

When people heal their cancer using natural treatments, it can be hard to know whether one thing did it or a combination of things. It is about "healing the body." I tend to think cancer is a disease. I think it is true that poisons like glyphosate (Roundup) give you cancer (the World Health Organization says it does), as do G5 wireless radiation, stress, and all the other poisons we ingest in our food and environment. So, it makes sense that if "dis-ease" causes cancer, you would use "ease" to cure it. No stress, no poisons, fresh organic food, fun, and laughter I say this because big pharma has so many writers in their employ writing disinformation to confuse people, and some natural treatments lack scientific evidence but have lots of anecdotal evidence.

I believe all the therapies in this book are in the "ease" category, and when combined—like the Japanese eat a wide range of foods to capture all their nutrient needs—with a myriad of protocols like organic food, clean water, rebound, B17, etc., it does not just target cancer; it targets your overall health so you can be at "ease" and your body will heal itself.

Dr. Keith Scott: Mommy from Las Vegas said it right. Your system can handle quite a bit of trash, but it has a tipping point. You should never get to the tipping point (cancer, heart attack, etc.), so you should eat 95% healthy every day. I frequently believe that junk food and laziness are unresolved issues from your childhood. Why wouldn't you have the most optimal diet to make yourself perfectly healthy unless there is some negative, even evil, thinking tucked away deep down inside of you?

So, choose your protocols based on where you live, what's at hand, and how much self-control you have or not.

Make sure you cut out at least five bad things. Sugar, 5G, glyphosate, laziness, and negative thinking, and adopt at least

5 good things. Organic food, pure mineralized water, love and happiness, turmeric with a pinch of black pepper, and exercise Finally, it makes sense to try and kill cancer directly, like with B17 and mistletoe, as well as boost your immune system so it can kill it too.

Thank you for purchasing this small book

roditch@protonmail.com